101 CASTOR OIL USES, RECIPES AND HEALING

By Czech J. Kimberly

Table of Contents

Introduction

Castor oil is made from the seeds of the castor bean plant, which grows in some eastern countries. The oil comes from pressing the seeds of the castor bean plant. Castor oil has a lot of ricinoleic acid, which is a type of fatty acid that helps reduce inflammation, fights against harmful substances in the body, and reduces pain.

Castor oil has been used as a natural remedy for a very long time. Ancient Egyptians used castor oil to help dry eyes feel better and to help with constipation. In Ayurvedic medicine, which is a type of medicine from India, castor oil is used to help with arthritis pain and treat skin problems.

Nowadays, castor oil is used in medicine, drugs, and factories. It can be found in a lot of soaps, makeup, and hair and skin products.

Castor oil can be used by either swallowing it or putting it on the skin, depending on what you want to use it for. Some people swallow it to help them poop or to bring on labor when they are pregnant. Others use the oil on their skin and hair to keep them moisturized.

Castor oil is good for your health in many ways because it has different healing properties like fighting germs, viruses, and helping wounds to heal.

The FDA doesn't control dietary supplements much, so they might not be right for you. Supplements can have different effects on people. These effects depend on factors such as what type of supplement it is, how much of it you take, how often you take it, and if you're taking any other medications. Before you start taking any supplements, please talk to your doctor or pharmacist.

"Safety worries"

Not everyone can use castor oil. Pregnant women should not use castor oil because it can make the womb squeeze.

It's also not a good idea for kids under 12 to use it regularly. Before giving your child castor oil, talk to their doctor.

In people over 60, using castor oil for a long time can make constipation worse. It can also decrease the level of potassium in your body.

You should not use castor oil if you are taking specific medicines.

Diuretics can lower the amount of potassium in your body. Antibiotics like tetracyclines, drugs for bones, blood thinners, and heart medicines can also have side effects. Castor oil not only tastes bad to many people, but it also has a lot of side effects. Just like other laxatives that make you go to the bathroom, this one can make your stomach hurt and give you diarrhea. It can also stop your body from absorbing nutrients from food.

Eases Trouble Going to the Bathroom

Castor oil is mainly known for helping with constipation when you can't poop. The oil helps the muscles push waste through the intestines so it can be removed from the body. The United States FDA says castor oil is a safe and effective laxative, but not many people use it anymore because there are better options with fewer side effects.

Castor oil can make it easier to go to the bathroom, make poop softer, and make it feel like you're completely finished going to the bathroom.

Castor oil can also be used to clean the bowels before medical tests, like colonoscopies, but doctors usually use different kinds of laxatives for this.

Castor oil usually makes you poop within six to 12 hours after you take it.

Has the ability to keep skin from getting dry.
Castor oil is full of fatty acids and can keep your skin moisturized and healthy. Castor oil keeps your skin soft and smooth by locking in moisture. Like other oils that are good for the skin, castor oil also helps to stop moisture from leaving the skin.

Companies put castor oil in things like lotions, lip balms, and makeup to make them moisturizing and keep your skin hydrated.

Castor oil can be used by itself to keep your skin hydrated. However, it is very concentrated, so you might want to mix it with carrier oil (like almond, coconut, or jojoba oil) before putting it on your face and body.

There is not a lot of research on how castor oil helps skin. Studies show that the fatty acids in castor oil can help heal skin and make acne scars, fine lines, and wrinkles look less noticeable. However, we need to do more research to fully understand the impact.

Keep Dentures Clean
Dentures need to be cleaned every day to keep plaque from building up and to keep the mouth healthy. This will also help to keep the whole body healthy. Plaque is a

thin, sticky layer of bacteria and fungi that often forms on false teeth. People who wear dentures are more likely to get oral fungal infections, especially Candida (yeast), which can build up on dentures and increase the risk of denture stomatitis, a painful infection in the mouth.

Studies show that castor oil can fight bacteria and fungus, which can help keep dentures clean. A study showed that soaking dentures in a 10% castor oil solution for 20 minutes can kill oral bacteria and fungi. Another research discovered that cleaning dentures and soaking them in castor oil can help decrease Candida infections in people who wear dentures.

Helps Induce Labor in Pregnancy

Castor oil is an old way to help start labor. This used to be the most popular way to start labor, and some midwives still like to use it to help start labor.

Castor oil can make you go to the bathroom, and some people think this helps start labor. When you swallow castor oil, it makes your bowels work, which can upset the uterus and make it contract. Castor oil also helps make more prostaglandins, which are fats that act like hormones and help get the cervix ready for childbirth.

A study in 2018 found that almost 91% of pregnant women who took castor oil to start their labor were able to have a vaginal birth without any problems. A study of 19 others found that taking castor oil by mouth is a safe and effective way to get the cervix ready for vaginal birth and to start labor.

Taking castor oil to start labor can cause bad side effects like feeling sick, throwing up, and having diarrhea. Some doctors advise not to use castor oil to start labor because it can make the baby pass its first poop before being born, which could be dangerous. Do not take castor oil to start labor unless your doctor tells you to do so.

For Arthritis pain.
Castor oil may help reduce joint pain caused by arthritis because it can reduce inflammation.

An old study found that taking castor oil may help lessen knee pain caused by osteoarthritis. In the experiment, the people took castor oil pills three times a day for four weeks. At the end of the study, 92% of people with osteoarthritis said their pain got much better, and they didn't have any bad side effects.

Researchers looked at using castor oil on the skin to see if it helps with joint pain. Participants in the study rubbed castor oil onto the skin above their sore knees once a day for two weeks. The scientists found that castor oil helped to reduce joint pain and swelling.

How Castor Oil helps to make hair healthy

You may have heard that castor oil can help hair grow or stop it from falling out. But, there is no proof from science to confirm this.

You may have also heard that castor oil can help with dandruff and make itchy scalps feel better. Some dandruff products have castor oil, but there is no proof that castor oil alone can treat dandruff well. There are some things that make hair healthy where castor oil could work well.

Some people put castor oil on their hair to keep it from getting dry. This is because castor oil can make hair shiny and prevent split ends and breakage by keeping it well-lubricated.

Castor oil can help protect your scalp and hair from infections because it has properties that fight bacteria and fungus and reduce swelling.

Is it okay to use Castor Oil
Castor oil is usually safe in small amounts, but can be harmful in larger amounts. If you take too much castor oil by mouth, it can cause an overdose. Signs of taking too much castor oil include: - Nausea - Vomiting - Diarrhea - Abdominal pain - Dehydration.

- Stomach pain

- Diarrhea is when you have bowel movements that are loose and watery.
- Feeling unsteady or lightheaded
- Feeling very dizzy and passing out.
- Feeling sick to your stomach.
- Breathing trouble
- Tight feeling in the throat

Since castor oil can make muscles move, some people should not use it.

Pregnant people should not use the oil unless a doctor says it's okay during labor because it could cause early contractions.

People, who have problems with their stomach and intestines, like inflammatory bowel disease.

People who have stomach pain that could be from a blocked intestine, a hole in the intestine, or an inflamed appendix.

Castor oil is safe to put on your skin, but it could cause an allergic reaction in some people. This might make your skin red, swollen, itchy, or give you a rash. Try a little bit of oil on a small part of your skin first to make sure it doesn't cause any problems before using it on more of your skin.

You could get an allergic reaction after using the oil.

A fast look over
Castor oil is a type of oil that comes from squeezing the seeds of the castor bean plant. You can either swallow the oil or put it on your skin or hair.

For a long time, people have used castor oil to make themselves look better and to help with many different health problems. Castor oil can help with reducing inflammation, protecting against damage from harmful molecules, fighting fungal infections, and relieving pain which can be good for your health. It can help you poop, make your skin not dry, clean fake teeth, and start a baby coming out. There is not a lot of research that shows that castor oil might help with joint pain, but we need more research to be sure.

Many people say that castor oil can make hair, eyelashes, and eyebrows grow, but there is no proof that it actually works.

Drinking castor oil can make your stomach hurt, give you diarrhea, and make you feel sick. When you put castor oil on your skin, it can make you have an allergy. You might get red, itchy, and swollen skin. While many people think castor oil is safe, it may not be safe for everyone. Before you use castor oil as a natural remedy, talk to a healthcare provider first.

How to Use Castor Oil on Your Skin: Simple DIY Recipes

Castor oil is very popular in the clean beauty industry because it has lots of good things in it like antioxidants, proteins, vitamin E, and healthy fatty acids. It also gets into the skin easily and keeps water out, which helps it keep skin moist.

You can use castor oil at home for different purposes like cleaning your face, moisturizing your skin, making body scrubs, and for giving massages.

Castor oil is created by squashing the beans of the Ricinus communis plant and taking out the oil from inside. The product is thick and has a yellow color compared to other vegetable oils.

Castor oil lasts a long time and stays liquid in hot and cold temperatures. It is good for beauty products because it stays the same consistency.

Cleanser and makeup remover made from castor oil for your face.

Castor oil is thick, so mix it with a lighter oil before putting it on your face.

To make an oil cleanser, mix one spoon of castor oil with one spoon of grapeseed or sweet almond oil.

To take off makeup, use your fingers to put the oil mix on your face, and rub it in well. Be kind and giving, but don't overdo it.

Next, use a damp part of a washcloth or an organic cotton makeup remover pad, and gently wipe it across your skin. Keep doing this until all the makeup is gone and the cloth or pad is clean.

Cleaning your skin with oil should remove all the dirt and makeup. You can wash your face first, or just use toner and moisturizer.

Nighttime facial serum made from castor oil

Ingredients

- 1 spoon of argan oil
- 1 spoonful of castor oil
- 1 small spoon of oil from rosehip seeds

- Geranium oil extracted from geranium plants.

Instructions

To make an easy and very moisturizing face serum, mix argan oil, castor oil, and rosehip seed oil in a small container and shake it.

Put a few drops of geranium oil and mix it again for a nice, clean smell.

Apply the serum to your face before going to sleep, after you have cleaned and toned your skin. This serum is thick, so it's better to use it at night. It might feel too heavy during the day or when you wear makeup.

Body scrub with sugar and castor oil

You can make expensive sugar body scrubs at home using castor oil and a few other ingredients.

- Get a small glass jar or any other container and put one cup of regular white sugar in it. You can also use brown sugar if you have it, but don't use powdered sugar.
- Next, pour 1/4 cup of castor oil little by little and mix it with the sugar. You can fill the cup with white sugar, but if you want it to be more runny, you can add more oil. If you want it less wet, use less oil (or add a little more sugar).
- Once you get the thickness you like, put in your favorite

scented oils. Orange and lemon can make you feel happy, while lavender and ylang-ylang can make you feel calm and peaceful.

Be sure to cover your sugar mix to keep it dry. If water gets in, the sugar will dissolve and you'll have a messy liquid.

Gentle, Calming Massage Oil

Ingredients

- 3 tablespoons of castor oil
- Lavender oil
- Bergamot oil made from bergamot oranges
- Chamomile oil made from chamomile flowers.

Instructions

You can make a relaxing massage oil for tense shoulders and a sore neck by mixing castor oil with a few drops of lavender, bergamot, and chamomile essential oils. Combine in a bottle and shake it thoroughly.

To use the aromatic oil, put a few drops on your hands and then rub it on your shoulders and neck. This will help you relax before going to bed.

Commonly Asked Questions

Does castor oil clog pores.

Castor oil has a rating of one on the comedogenic scale, which goes from zero to five. It might clog pores a little and works well on oily and older skin.

How can you tell if the castor oil is good for the environment.

Castor oil comes from a natural plant, but sometimes the plant is sprayed with harmful chemicals which can pollute the air, land, and water. Be sure to buy organic and non-GMO castor oil to make sure it's sustainable.

Castor oil helps with poop problems.
Castor oil is a type of liquid that you can drink. People usually take it during the day because it works fast.

- Adults should take 15 ml of castor oil to treat constipation.

To make it tasteless strong, put castor oil in the fridge for an hour to cool it down. Next, pour it into a tall glass full of juice and mix it together. You can buy castor oil that has flavors added to it.

Castor oil works fast. You will notice changes in 2 to 6 hours after taking it. Since castor oil works fast, it's not a good idea to take it before going to bed, like you would with other laxatives.

Just like other strong laxatives, it's not good to take castor oil for a long time. Over time, it can make your intestines weaker and lead to long-lasting constipation. If you keep having trouble going to the bathroom, go see your doctor.

Castor oil is a strong way to decrease inflammation and keep your mouth healthy. Taking good care of our teeth means trying out different dental products like toothpaste and mouthwash to keep them healthy. However, hidden in the history of old-fashioned treatments is a powerful medicine that hasn't been used much for taking care of teeth.

This amazing natural product comes from the seeds of the Ricinus communis plant. It has many benefits for the gums and teeth, especially because it is really good at reducing inflammation.

Exploring Castor Oil's Ability to Reduce Inflammation
The main reason castor oil is good for you is because it contains ricinoleic acid, which is a type of healthy fat. This part makes up 90% of castor oil and is known for its ability to reduce swelling.

The importance of inflammation in keeping your mouth healthy.

Inflammation is how the body reacts to things that can hurt it, like injuries or infections. In the mouth, inflammation often makes your gums red and swollen. It's a common sign of gum disease. If not treated, inflammation can cause gums to shrink, spaces between teeth and gums, and even teeth to fall out.

Treating swollen gums with direct action

When you put castor oil on your skin, it goes into your gums and delivers ricinoleic acid to the right place. This helps to soothe angry cells, makes pain go away and lessens redness.

Some germs in the mouth let out poisons that can bother the gums, making them swollen and sore. Castor oil has natural germ-fighting abilities that can help reduce gum swelling by getting rid of harmful bacteria.

Improving the flow of blood in your body

Good blood flow is really important for keeping your gums healthy. Castor oil helps blood flow better, so the body's defense cells can get to the problem areas faster and help them heal.

Healthy gums are important for having healthy teeth. When your gums are swollen, it can weaken the support for your teeth. Castor oil reduces swelling and pain.

Stops gums from moving back.

Castor oil stops gums from moving away from the teeth and exposing the sensitive root area by controlling inflammation. Inflammation can cause gaps between the gums and teeth where bad bacteria can grow. By reducing swelling, castor oil helps prevent pockets from forming, which keeps the teeth and bone safe.

Strengthens the natural protection of teeth.
In a healthy mouth, saliva helps protect it from germs. It balances acids and removes food bits. Castor oil helps keep your mouth healthy by controlling inflammation. This makes sure

that saliva can protect your teeth
from getting decay.

How to Use Castor Oil for a Healthy Mouth

Gum massage is when you gently
rub and stimulate the gums with
your fingers or a special tool to
keep them healthy.

Every night, put a little castor oil
on your fingers and rub it onto
your gums before you go to sleep.
This practice helps the oil work
better and also helps blood move
through the body.

Oil pulling is a natural remedy for
cleaning your mouth and
improving oral health. It involves
swishing oil around in your mouth
for a few minutes and then spitting

it out. This can help remove harmful bacteria and improve the condition of your teeth and gums.

Oil pulling is usually done with sesame or coconut oil, but you can also use castor oil. Swish one tablespoon of oil in your mouth for 15-20 minutes and then spit it out. This method removes harmful substances from the body and decreases swelling.

Boost your toothpaste
Put a little bit of castor oil in your regular toothpaste before you brush your teeth. This little extra thing can make your toothbrushing routine even better at reducing inflammation.

In conclusion, castor oil is very helpful for taking care of your teeth and mouth. Its strong ability to reduce inflammation is really good for your gums and teeth. It's a very important part of keeping your mouth healthy. Always make sure to use 100% pure castor oil that is cold-pressed and doesn't contain any hexane to get all the benefits.

Using Castor Oil to Start Labor

Castor oil is a type of oil that has been used for helping start labor, but we don't know much about if it is really safe or if it really works. Some studies say drinking castor oil can help start labor for some women, but it can also make you vomit and feel sick. It can also be bad for the baby. It's a good idea to talk to your doctor before using castor oil to help start labor.

Castor oil is a type of oil that comes from the seeds of the castor plant. It is in many things that are made, like soap, oil, plant food, and paint. Castor oil is sometimes used as a medicine to help with constipation. For many years, castor oil has been used to help start labor, but there is not much evidence to prove that it actually works.

Can I use castor oil to start labor?

Using castor oil to try to make labor start can be dangerous, and there is no certainty that it will actually work. Studies on castor oil's ability to start labor have had different results, and it could make you have diarrhea, feel sick, throw up, and might cause stress for your baby. It's important to talk to your doctor before trying natural methods to start labor.

Several small studies have shown that castor oil can help start labor in some women. A study of 50 pregnant women who were overdue found that those who took castor oil were more likely to go into labor within 24 hours compared to those who didn't take castor oil. A small study showed that castor oil helped to start labor in women who had given birth before, but not in women having their first baby. An earlier study of around 200 women with early water breaking showed that those who took castor oil went into labor faster. At the same time, a study with mice showed that an important part of castor oil makes the intestines and uterine muscles work harder, which releases prostaglandins and can cause contractions.

However, a big study of over 600 women in southeast Asia did not find any proof that castor oil helps start labor.

Research on the possible problems from using castor oil is not clear yet. The research in southeast Asia found that castor oil is safe for women and their babies.

However, some other research shows that women who use castor oil to start labor may feel sick afterward. They might throw up or have diarrhea. A study on castor oil found that it may cause babies to pass their first stool before they are born, which can be harmful to their health.

How much castor oil should I use?

There isn't a set amount of castor oil to use for starting labor. Actually, experts can't decide if it's safe to use castor oil to start labor.

Research on using castor oil to start labor usually involves drinking a one-time dose of 60 milliliters, which is about 4 tablespoons, when a person is 40 or 41 weeks pregnant. Castor oil is usually mixed with juice or another liquid to hide its bad taste. It's best to take castor oil when you haven't eaten anything.

Don't use castor oil before bed because it might make you have to go to the bathroom a lot and feel sick.

How long does it take for castor oil to start working?
There isn't enough proof that castor oil will help start labor. But one research found that women who used castor oil to start labor were more likely to go into labor within 24 hours than women who didn't use it.

Is it okay to drink castor oil when you're pregnant.
It's not a good idea to drink castor oil before 40 weeks of pregnancy because it might cause early labor to start. Do not use castor oil for constipation when you are pregnant. Before using castor oil

to start labor when you are close to giving birth, talk to your doctor first.

Possible problems from using castor oil to induce labor

Taking castor oil to start labor has many dangers. Castor oil is a powerful medicine that makes you go to the bathroom, and if you eat it, it can cause:

Feeling sick to your stomach

"Diarrhea" means having loose or watery stools, often with frequent bowel movements.

Muscle pain or discomfort.

Dehydration means your body doesn't have enough water.

Low blood pressure means that
the force of blood against the walls
of your arteries is lower than it
should be.

Feeling like you are spinning or
unsteady.

Taking castor oil to start labor
might make your baby have a
bowel movement before birth,
which could cause problems
sometimes.

29 Amazing Ways to Use and Benefit from Castor Oil

For a long time, doctors and traditional healers have used castor oil because it has many health benefits. Many people believe that the ancient Egyptians were the first to find out about the different ways to use and the advantages of castor oil.

Many people think that Cleopatra used a light yellow liquid to make the whites of her eyes look brighter. Castor oil is easy to use and is gentle on your skin, so it's great for treating a lot of different health problems.

Advantages of Castor Oil
Castor oil is a light yellow vegetable oil made from crushing castor oil plant seeds. Many of the good things about using castor oil come from the way it is made. Castor oil is a kind of fat that is mostly made up of ricinoleic acid, which is a type of unsaturated fat.

- Skin problems/maladies
- Reliefs constipation problems
- Support for the body's defense system
- Reduces swelling and pain.
- Kills germs
- Acts as Lymphatic stimulant

Castor oil has been used for a long time to help with skin problems, infections, constipation, and making hair healthier. Recent research has found that castor oil can help the immune system and act as an anti-inflammatory, antimicrobial, and lymphatic stimulant.

You can use castor oil in a few different ways. Put it on your skin, make a castor oil pack with it, or mix it with other oils to use it on your skin as a remedy. You can mix it into milk or warm water, or take it as a supplement.

1. A natural way to help with arthritis pain

Castor oil can help reduce inflammation, making it a good oil for massaging achy joints, sore muscles, and irritated nerves. Castor oil has something called ricinoleic acid in it, which can help reduce inflammation in the body. This makes it a safe treatment for arthritis pain. Here are different ways you can use castor oil to help with arthritis pain.

Instructions

- Take a piece of natural cotton flannel fabric and fold it to make three or four layers.
- Soak the area in castor oil and put it on the sore joints.
- Cover the cloth with plastic wrap and place a warm heating pad or hot water bottle on top of the area. Let it sit for 45 minutes.
- Do this every day to help lessen pain and swelling in your joints.

- The plastic wrap will stop the heating pad or water bottle from getting greasy.
- Put the pads in a Ziploc bag and keep them in the fridge until you want to use them again.
- Take the castor oil by mouth, mix with your favorite drink.
- Rub warm castor oil onto the sore joints. To help your skin absorb the product better, rub it into your skin before bedtime and keep it on all night.
- To prevent burning the skin, make sure the castor oil is not too hot when putting it on the sore area.
- To help with bad arthritis pain, put a little bit of ginger powder into a cup of hot water. After the water gets

cold, put in two spoons of castor oil. Make sure to stir the drink well before you drink it.

This treatment works best if you drink it when you first wake up or right before you go to bed.

If you don't like the taste of castor oil, you can take a pill instead. However, this won't work as well as pure castor oil.

2. How to Remove Stretch Marks

Stretch marks are lines on the skin that can happen when the body changes quickly, like during pregnancy or when someone gains or loses weight fast. They can also happen as the body gets older, when hormones are not balanced, or when the skin swells. Castor oil is really good for fixing many skin problems. The lotion has lots of good stuff in it, like fatty acids, which make it great for keeping your skin moist and getting rid of stretch marks.

- Use your fingers to rub castor oil on the stretch marks until the whole area is covered.
- To make your skin more moisturized, mix 2 tablespoons of coconut or almond oil with 1 tablespoon of castor oil.
- Do not put the treatment on skin that is cut or hurt.
- Cover the area with a thin cotton cloth.

- Keep the cloth on the area for 15-20 minutes so the oil can go deep inside.
- Using a heating pad or hot water bottle on the area will make it heal faster.
- Keep doing this regularly to make your stretch marks look a lot smaller.

3. Using Castor Oil to Treat Acne

Acne happens when dirt and oil clog your skin pores, making them irritated and swollen. "Most acne treatments have benzoyl peroxide and salicylic acid, which can make the skin dry. " Castor oil, like neem oil, is a natural ingredient that can clean your skin by removing dirt, dead skin cells, extra oils, and bacteria without making your skin dry.

Follow these instructions

- Put a bowl of hot water on a steady table and get a towel.
- Put the towel over your head and lean over the water bowl.
- By doing this, your pores open up, and the castor oil can go deep into your skin.
- Put your face above the bowl for a few minutes.
- Get a washcloth wet with warm water and put a small amount of castor oil on it.
- Use only a dime-sized amount of oil.

- Gently use the washcloth to clean the sore area.
- When you put the castor oil on, move your finger in small circles.
- Leave the castor oil on your skin for the whole night.
- When you wake up, use a wet towel to remove the castor oil from your skin.
- Splash your face with cold water a few times.
- Cold water makes your pores smaller, and warm water makes your pores bigger.
- Gently dry your skin and use a facial cleanser to remove the rest of the castor oil.

For good results, do these steps every day for 10 to 14 days. You can use castor oil a few times a week to stop acne.

4. Strong face cleaner

In addition to helping with acne, you can also use castor oil to clean your face deeply. Instead of using strong chemicals that can make your skin dry, you can use castor oil as a cleanser to quickly get rid of pimples and clean your skin deeply. It will remove dirt, bacteria, dead skin cells, and extra oils while keeping your skin soft and smooth.

Instructions

- Rub a lot of the oil mixture in your hand, and then rub your hands together to make the oil warm.
- Gently rub the oil into your face using slow and steady

movements. Focus on any areas that need extra care.

- When your pores are full of water, use a clean towel soaked in hot water.
- Put the cloth on your face. Keep it on until it feels cool.
- Gently use the washcloth to clean your face, then rinse it in hot water.
- Do these steps over and over again to really clean your face.
- Make sure you don't scrub your face too hard at the end.

5. Getting rid of small lines and folds in the skin (Wrinkles).

Castor oil is good for making wrinkles and fine lines less

because it goes deep into your skin and helps make more elastin and collagen. These two parts in the skin make it stretchy and firm. Castor oil makes your skin smooth and soft. It helps your face to stay moisturized and give it a fuller look. This also helps to make fine lines and wrinkles less noticeable. To make the most of the castor oil treatment, do these steps.

Here's how to get there

- Wash your face with your regular face wash and cold water.
- Dry your skin by gently patting it with a towel.
- Use a cotton ball soaked in toner to wipe off any leftover cleaner.

- If you don't have toner, you can use rose water or witch hazel instead.
- Let the toner dry, then put a little castor oil in your hand and rub your hands together to warm up the oil.
- Gently rub the oil on your face in small circles.
- Do the same thing every day.
- For best results, put the oil on your face before going to sleep at night.

6. Using castor oil can help your hair to grow.

Castor oil, especially Jamaican Black Castor oil, is now used a lot for making hair grow healthier and thicker. When you use it on your scalp often, it can help your hair grow, protect against damage from styling and products, make your hair shiny and thick, prevent dry scalp, and make your hair healthier overall. When you put castor oil on the tips of your hair, it can make your hair less frizzy and fix split ends. Follow these steps to make your hair stronger and grow it longer.

Instructions

- Put castor oil on your scalp and roots with your fingertips.
- Make sure to spread it evenly on your head.
- Avoid getting oil in your hair. Because it is thick, it can be hard to take off.

- Put a plastic cap on your hair and then wrap a towel around your head.
- Leave the oil on your hair for at least fifteen minutes.
- For the best outcome, leave it in overnight.
- To get rid of the castor oil, wash your hair well with shampoo.
- For best results, do this every week for 6-8 weeks.

7. Alleviating trouble going to the bathroom.

Many people use castor oil to help them poop when they are constipated. The different parts of the natural remedy for constipation work like a strong medicine that helps you go to the bathroom. It makes both the small

and large intestines work better
and clears out your colon, so that
any stuck poop can move through.
The fatty acids in castor oil help
the bowel to hold onto its moisture
and make it easier for things to
pass through. (Read more about
using Castor oil to treat
constipation)

To use castor oil for constipation
relief, just follow these steps.

**Recipe for using castor oil to
relieve constipation.**

- 30 to 60 grams of Castor Oil
- Warm milk or water
- A glass container made of
  glass.
- Ginger (You can choose to
  add it or not)

Instructions

- Mix 30 to 60 grams of castor oil into a glass of warm milk.
- Replace milk with a glass of warm water if you don't like it.
- Finish all the drink in the glass.
- If the mixture smells too strong, you can put some ginger in it.
- In about an hour, you will start to feel the castor oil working.

8. Makes your body stronger to fight off sickness

Regularly using castor oil is thought to help improve different parts of the immune system, like how the lymphatic system works, the health of the thymus gland, and how blood moves through the body. Lymphocytes are a kind of white blood cell in the body's defense system. They fight against things that can harm the body, like bacteria and toxins. Castor oil helps the body make the right amount of lymphocytes, which are stored in the lymph nodes, thymus gland, and tissue in the small intestine. Put castor oil packs on your stomach to help your body soak up the oil better.

9. Treating Ringworm

Ringworm is a skin condition caused by a fungus that makes a red rash in the shape of a ring.

Research has found that almost 1 in 5 people have had ringworm at least one time in their life. Even though it can be bothersome, castor oil is a great way to treat ringworm. The undecylenic acid in castor oil can kill fungal infections.

10.   Reduce how scars look

Castor oil is really good for making scars look smaller or stopping them from forming. The oil's fatty acids help the body's lymphatic system and prevent scars. While it can't make scars go away completely, it can make them look better.

11.   Treat rough, dry heels.

Castor oil is great for dry skin and can help heal cracked heels. It has lots of vitamins and important nutrients that help moisturize dry, cracked skin. Just massage castor oil onto your feet, wear socks, and leave it overnight. You will see a big change.

12.   Start labor

Castor oil can help start labor. When you swallow castor oil, it helps make your bowels move. Castor oil can cause the uterus to get irritated and start having contractions. Please take a look at the extra details provided.

13.   Treat Sunburn

Castor oil can help relieve sunburn pain, and it feels cool like aloe. Ricinoleic acid helps prevent blisters from getting infected and reduces inflammation caused by sunburns.

14.   Use Castor Oil to make your eyebrows thicker.

Castor oil can help make your hair grow faster and stronger. Did you know that castor oil can make your eyebrows thicker. It has good stuff in it like antioxidants and vitamins that help make your eyebrow hair healthy and stop bacteria from stopping them growing.

15. **Make your eyelashes longer with castor oil**.

Castor oil has vitamins, proteins, and minerals that can make your eyelashes stronger and longer if you use it regularly. It also has antibacterial properties. When you put it on your skin, it goes deep down and makes the area moisturized and refreshed. This helps your eyelashes grow faster and stops them from breaking.

16. **Get rid of moles and skin tags**.

When you mix castor oil with baking soda, it can help remove moles and skin tags. Just put the paste on the hurting area and then cover it with a bandage. Doing this every day for four to six weeks will get rid of the moles and skin tags.

Dry skin Dry skin is when your skin doesn't have enough moisture. It can feel tight, itchy, or rough.

Recipe for Using Castor Oil to Treat Dry Skin

- 1 tablespoon of castor oil.
- Use Sunflower or Extra Virgin Olive Oil (about 9 tablespoons).

Dry skin is when your skin feels tight, itchy, and can start to crack. Usually, you are more likely to have dry skin in the fall and winter when the air is drier. You may also notice it as you get older, because your body makes less oil.

In other words, there are some things you can do if you have dry skin. When you take a shower, use warm water instead of hot water because hot water takes away the oil on your skin. After you shower, gently pat your skin dry instead of rubbing it. Try washing yourself every other day instead of every day, use soap that has moisturizer in it, and put on lotion (also with moisturizer) right after you get out of the shower.

Recipe for making hair conditioner.

- Use 3 tablespoons of castor oil.
- One spoon of jojoba or argan oil.
- Juice from half a lemon, if necessary.

As I said before, castor oil is great for making hair grow. Even if you don't want to make your hair grow faster, you can use castor oil instead of conditioner.

Castor oil can help treat dandruff because it has things in it that can fight bacteria, fungi, and viruses. It makes frizzy hair and split ends less wild, and it adds moisture to your hair for a shiny look.

To make castor oil conditioner, mix castor oil with Jojoba or Argon oil. If you have dandruff, you can try using the juice from half a lemon along with your treatment.

Packs made with castor oil

- Use a piece of soft fabric like flannel, cotton, or wool.
- Soak in Castor oil
- Put it on the area that's hurt or not feeling well.
- After you're done, put it in a plastic bag with a zipper so you can use it again later.

How safe is it to use castor oil.

Your health problem, how old you are, and how much you weigh will decide how much castor oil you should take. Before you use castor oil, talk to your doctor to make sure you are taking the right amount.

Castor oil can be used in many different ways.

Castor oil is often used to help with constipation, but it can also help with other things. Castor oil can help your hair grow back and get stronger. It can also help with arthritis. There are many different ways that castor oil can be helpful. People have been using castor oil for a long time, and many people like it for its benefits.

17.   **Make cuticles softer and get rid of brittle nails.**

Castor oil has a lot of vitamin E, which is really good for nails that are dry and break easily. Rubbing it on your nails and the skin around them every night will make your cuticles soft and your nails look healthy.

Recipe for making fern plants healthier.

- 4 cups of hot water.
- One tablespoon of castor oil.

- Use just a little bit of baby shampoo.

18.   Revive Your Ferns

Castor oil can be used to make your ferns healthier. It has lots of minerals and vitamins that can help if your ferns don't look good. Mix the warm water, castor oil and baby shampoo together, and then pour a few drops of the mixture onto the soil. Make sure to water your ferns regularly, and in a few days, they will look healthy and strong again.

19.   Keep moles away from your yard.

If you have a problem with moles ruining your yard, castor oil might help you get rid of them. Combine

2 gallons of water with 1/2 cup of castor oil and then pour it into the holes where the moles are. The solution won't hurt the moles, it will just make it uncomfortable for them so they'll go somewhere else to dig.

20. Help the lymph system

Your lymphatic system helps remove waste from your body. If you have trouble with drains or things not flowing properly, castor oil can help fix the problem. Using castor oil packs on your lymph nodes helps your body to soak up the oil fast.

20.   Lessens skin
redness and swelling

Castor oil can help heal bug bites, rashes, and itches because it has strong antibacterial and anti-inflammatory powers. To reduce redness and swelling on the skin, just put some castor oil on a bandage and put it on the sore spot. To cover big areas, dip a cotton ball in castor oil and put it on the place that hurts. Wash it off after one hour, and do it again many times during the day.

21.   Treats toenail
infection.

The undecylenic acid in castor oil can help get rid of fungus in the body. Soak your feet in warm water with Epsom salt for five minutes to help cure toenail fungus. Put lots of castor oil on the toenail that is affected after soaking.

How to make lip balm using castor oil

- One teaspoon of castor oil
- One teaspoon of glycerin
- A few drops of lemon juice.

22.   Moisturizes dry lips.

The fatty acids in castor oil help to make dry, chapped lips moisturized and soft. Put castor oil on your lips a few times a day to make them soft and moist. You can make a calming cream by mixing castor oil, glycerin, and lemon juice. Put on before you go to sleep to keep dry lips moisturized.

23. Helps with the pain and discomfort of migraines.

Castor oil is a good way to make headaches and migraines feel better. To help with migraine and headache pain, gently massage a small amount of oil onto your forehead for one minute. You will start to feel the effects in two to three minutes.

24. Helps to decrease the pain during periods.

Rubbing warm castor oil on your stomach can help make menstrual cramps and period pain feel better. The acid in castor oil helps reduce swelling and is a pain reliever. Castor oil packs are great

for easing the pain of menstrual
cramps.

25. Ease the pain of mouth sores.

Castor oil is a good natural
treatment for mouth sores because
it fights bacteria and reduces
swelling. To help heal mouth
sores, put a little bit of castor oil or
peppermint oil on them. After a
few minutes, wash out your mouth
with water and do it several times
a day.

26. Relieve sore muscles and pain.

When you put it on your skin,
ricinoleic acid can go deeper and
help reduce inflammation in the
tissues. To feel better from achy

muscles, put a cloth soaked in castor oil on the hurting area and then use a warm pad or hot water bottle on top. The warmth helps to carry the castor oil to the swollen joints and tissue.

27.   Improve your sleep.

If you can't sleep, castor oil might help you fall asleep. Instead of taking strong and addictive medicine for your trouble sleeping, try rubbing castor oil on your eyelids before you go to sleep. Your body takes in the oil and helps your blood flow better, making you feel relaxed and aiding with sleep.

28.   Get rid of corns.

Corns on your feet can hurt and bother you. Castor oil helps to hydrate and remove them. To treat corns, put your feet in warm water for about fifteen minutes. Dry your feet and put castor oil on the corn. After about ten days of treatment, you should be able to remove the corns easily.

29.   Anti-Fungal Properties

Castor oil has a substance called undecylenic acid that can stop fungus from growing. The undecylenic acid in this natural remedy is good for many different fungal infections, like yeast infections, athlete's foot, and ringworm. Mix coconut oil with this and put it on the part of your body that is affected. Leave it on while you sleep and the fungus will get better.

Regular castor oil versus organic castor oil

People think Jamaican black castor oil is a very strong mixture. Jamaican castor oil is stronger because of the way they make it. Jamaican black castor oil is made by roasting and grinding organic seeds by hand, then boiling them to get 100% pure dark oil. It's different from regular castor oil.

When you cook beans for a long time, they will have more ash in them. When castor oil has a lot of ash in it, people think it works better because the ash makes the oil stronger. The more ash there is, the darker the oil looks.

How do we make Castor Oil

Castor oil is made by squeezing the seeds of the castor oil plant. The plant is very poisonous and has a toxic protein and alkaloid called ricin. To make castor oil, first take the beans from the castor oil plant and cook them. Then, squeeze the beans to let the oil out.

What are the bad effects of castor oil.

Castor oil is a natural medicine that is approved to use in small doses. However, if you take too much or use it for a long time, you may still have some mild to moderate symptoms.

Before using a lot of castor oil on your skin or taking it by mouth, check if you are allergic to it by doing a small test on a small area of your skin. Put a little bit of castor oil on your arm and leave it there for a day (24 hours). If your skin feels irritated or itchy, don't use castor oil.

When you use castor oil, be careful. If you take too much castor oil, it can make you very sick and cause serious health problems.

Further side effects include:

- Stomach pains
- Diarrhea

- Feeling sick
- Low blood pressure
- Difficulty with blood flow in the pelvic region
- Skin irritation
- Difficult breathing.

More Castor Oil Recipes

Recipe for using castor oil on oily skin.

- Three tablespoons of Castor Oil.
- Sunflower or Olive Oil (7 tablespoons)

Skin that produces too much oil.

Having oily skin can cause a few problems.

One issue is that oily skin can make your face look shiny, which some people might not like. Also, your face will feel greasy when you touch it.

Another issue is that the oil on your face can block your pores. When your skin's pores are blocked, you get acne. This makes your skin look bad and can cause permanent scars.

"Recipe for Using Castor Oil on Combin*ation Skin"

- Two tablespoons of castor oil.
- Sunflower or Extra Virgin Olive Oil (8 tablespoons)

Combination skin means your face has both oily and dry areas.

When you have combination skin, it means some parts of your face are dry and other parts are oily.

Many people have skin that is a combination of different types. The T-zone is the middle part of your face with your eyes, nose, and mouth. It's called that because it looks like a 'T'. The T-zone is the part of your face that gets oily, while the cheeks and under the eyes can be dry or flaky.

The way to treat combination skin is similar to treating oily skin, but with less castor oil and more sunflower (or extra virgin olive) oil.